PREGNANT PAUSE

PREGNANT PAUSE

10 Narratives of Pregnancy and Birth during the Global Pandemic

COURTNEY ELLISON MARSHALL, MPA

The stories in *Pregnant Pause* were gathered to give the women in the book a voice, provide support to women going through a similar experience in the future and document the historic time.

CONTENTS

INTRODUCTION

Strength is in community. It is with that sentiment that I started this project. As a woman who found out I was pregnant shortly before the COVID-19 lockdown swept the United States, I know the truth of that phrase all too well. Navigating uncharted waters in your own body while the outside world has turned upside down is a notable experience. Inner strength and resiliency are put to the test. One of the things we look for as humans, the support of others, was in scarce supply—along with toilet paper—for those who did not live the experience, the rest of us remember this part vividly.

The concept that social support has a positive impact on health is widely agreed upon.[i] One of my favorite studies involves a very basic and visual scientific experiment.[ii] Individual perceptions of a steep hill were measured with social support and without. More specifically, individuals who had a friend physically stand next to them, versus those who were left to perceive the steep hill alone, found the hill to be less steep. Similarly, those who thought of a friend during an imagery task versus those who thought of someone neutral or someone they disliked perceived the hill to be less steep. If the experience of being pregnant during the COVID-19 pandemic were a hill, it might as well be Mount Everest.

While I pride myself on my inner strength, I couldn't help but find comfort in the words of an elderly woman, Anita Sampson, who was a baby in a prior pandemic.[iii] Anita spoke of the strength her own mother had in a prior pandemic, and of the strength we all possessed to get through this pandemic. When Anita was finished speaking, words flashed on the television screen that highlighted the theme that new moms in quarantine were not alone.

Given the probability of future pandemics,[iv] it makes sense to build that community of strength now for the women who are pregnant during a pandemic or similar event in the future. To those women, I hope this book can serve as a pillar of strength, knowing there is a community of women who have come before you, standing with you.

The sentence, "Being pregnant during a global pandemic is …," can take so many different turns. It is truly a wild card of the game fill-in-the-blank. There are so many micro-experiences affecting this unique journey that it is impossible to "box" this experience in. The COVID-19 pandemic's direct and indirect implications were far-reaching with many aspects of life disrupted, often in an abrupt manner.

There were changes in the health care setting, in the workplace, and in everyday life at home. During the COVID-19 pandemic (particularly the early days), ob-gyn appointments and even delivery often excluded any support partners. As was published in July 2020 in JAMA Psychiatry, "This bewildering experience increases fear and alienation for women in labor and may increase risk for birth-related posttraumatic stress disorder, especially for women with preexisting trauma … having a partner, supportive family member, or continuously present birth professional is known to improve psychological and obstetric outcomes for women in labor and their newborns."[v] Routine appointments themselves were sometimes reduced or moved to telehealth and concrete information on COVID-19 itself was lacking.[vi] There was also a spike in domestic violence throughout the world, including in the US.[vii] The risk of depression in pregnant women almost doubled compared to pre-pandemic risk.[viii] Amid layoffs and increasing childcare responsibilities[ix] the title of this September 2020 BLS Monthly Labor Review summary headline seems to have said it all: "COVID-19 recession is tougher on women."[x] Even the seemingly trivial but important milestones in many of our pregnancies, the in-person announcements and baby showers, were often canceled.[xi] The old Roman theory of "bread and circuses" was half applied during COVID-19 in the form of stimulus checks, but the celebratory circuses were purposely left out.

Amid the unwelcome changes and disruptions—meant to save lives and keep the health care system afloat—there were some things made easier by the "new normal." As many pregnant women will tell you, being in close proximity to a couch, bathroom, or refrigerator is preferred more often than not. For many, this was made a reality during the early COVID days when lockdowns were prevalent,[xii] and commutes were virtually nonexistent. Rules around work attire suddenly became more flexible (and pregnancy-friendly). Athleisure sales soared, with some claiming an 84 percent increase in orders since the pandemic began.[xiii] Pants with stretch waistbands quickly became the accepted workday attire for many newly remote workers.

Sharing, if nothing else, may help heal a post-COVID society. As was said in the early 2021 article, "How to heal the 'mass trauma' of COVID-19," "When it (trauma) goes unprocessed, undiscussed, perhaps actively repressed, the group's social tissues remain disturbed and unhealed. Individual trauma builds up unrecognised and festers under the cracks."[xiv] The same sentiment was echoed in 2023 by the American Psychological Association's chief executive officer, Arthur C. Evans Jr., PhD: "We cannot ignore the fact that we have been significantly changed by the loss of more than one million Americans, as well as the shift in our workplaces, school systems, and culture at large. To move toward posttraumatic growth, we must first identify and understand the psychological wounds that remain."[xv]

The last few paragraphs, filled with academic facts, shed light on the experience of being pregnant/newly postpartum during COVID-19, yet the best way to communicate the effects—mental, physical, logistical—is to share the stories of women who have lived it. I have filled these pages with their words, their thoughts, and their strength. To the women who experienced one of the most sacred yet common human conditions in a very abnormal time, I hope this book gives you a voice to express some of what you felt, learned, and endured.

MARISA'S STORY

I remember seeing news footage of police officers in China basically rounding up people with COVID in the early months of 2020. Must be kind of serious, my husband and I thought. Still, we never imagined that within a month, it would be next door and rock our lives. I was due with our first child, a boy, in mid-May 2020. Looking back now, it's a bit of a blur.

The impacts started with more of the normal things—stocking up on groceries and household items, grocery stores being wiped out. We canceled our baby shower around the time that travel was being restricted. I remember feeling like, "OK, another life chapter that isn't really going to plan"—as I'd been diagnosed with breast cancer when I was engaged, and we'd ended up having to move our wedding date, and I got married in a wig. There was some sorrow and self-pity there, but we kept our sense of perspective and moved on. The whole world was dealing with this sort of thing. A canceled baby shower wasn't the end of the world.

In late March though, the effects of COVID went from almost bemusing and hypothetical to very real. My father-in-law had attended a conference in Vegas in mid-March, when some of our elected officials were still saying the virus wasn't here, that there were very few cases, "soon to be 0." He became sick a few days later, and it was bad enough within a week of his return that he got tested at a drive-through COVID testing site. A couple days later, he received a positive result. My husband and sister-in-law left him Gatorade and soup, thinking he'd just have to ride out a rough cold for a while. My husband saw him at the gas pumps at some point around then but didn't want to go near him because he didn't want to get sick, especially with me being pregnant.

Within a day of the positive result, my husband received a phone call from his father's longtime girlfriend. She had been on the phone with his dad and said that he'd had trouble speaking due to difficulty breathing and was having such a hard time breathing that he couldn't keep a thermometer in with his mouth closed long enough to take his temperature. She was worried. I was trying to understand what was happening secondhand, as my husband was on the phone.

After he got off the phone, he called for an ambulance and went over to his father's house, wearing a hazmat type suit he had from volunteering with the fire department. He had to help carry his father, who couldn't walk, out of the house on a blanket. He was grey in the face and not really able to speak. My husband followed the ambulance to a local hospital, where they quickly determined he needed to go to a bigger hospital. A few hours later, he was put into a coma and intubated at that other hospital. My husband had a friend drop off some framed pictures from our house at the hospital entrance; even though his father was in a coma, you still wanted to do stuff like that. What else could we do? No one was allowed in the hospital. His dad was alone, with the medical staff.

Over the days that followed, my husband fielded terrible calls from doctors and nurses. Within the first day, a doctor was asking about "do not resuscitate" orders and saying it didn't look good. We kept up hope the best we could. I wasn't OK, but I tried to be strong for my husband. I cooked and hugged him and called friends and relatives with updates so he wouldn't have to.

We had a couple of "video calls" with nurses in hazmat suits and my father-in-law, who was in a coma, with tubes and everything else all over.

And, six days after my father-in-law entered the hospital, he died. Age sixty-six, one of the first COVID deaths in Maine.

A couple of weeks later, my water broke, three weeks early. We'll never know why, and it may have had nothing to do with it, but I know I was under severe stress in the weeks leading up to that.

When I was in labor, I kept having nightmarish visions of my father-in-law. I love my son and was so happy and grateful to have him, but it was not a happy time in our lives. It was tragic and nightmarish, surreal. The juxtaposition of life and death was overwhelming. When our son had some lung issues with being born a bit early, the terminology triggered some sort of PTSD—it was some of the same wording used to describe my father-in-law's failing body a few weeks earlier. I was bracing for terrible news, again.

My father-in-law missed meeting our son, his first grandchild, by just nineteen days. There was so much pain in 2020 for us. We were more isolated because of COVID ... so, normally you'd go hug your mother, your father's partner, your sister, and others after your dad died. My husband couldn't, not without risking infection, especially with more vulnerable people—like his mother who had been diagnosed with cancer recently.

We couldn't have a wake or funeral, for some kind of closure, because of that risk. Especially with many anticipated guests being in their sixties and older, we absolutely would not chance getting anyone else sick. So, we didn't get that closure, that celebration of life. We had the sudden, surreal loss of a giant in our lives, and ashes.

We also had to watch friends and family members, and the world at large, share memes mocking the virus, downplaying it, saying it was a hoax. We had to hear elected officials do the same. I was filled with feelings of hurt, rage, and protectiveness of my husband who had lost his dad to this.

But, despite the tragic and painful context of his birth, our son, Del, gave us so much strength in those early months. He kept us from crumbling. He kept us going. The world whirled around us, the pain and anger came … but we had our son. He would bring us so much joy in the months and years ahead.

I think for my husband, taking care of our son was a way to pay tribute to his own father. As he got a bit older, my husband took him in his father's Jeep, or on his excavator. I think it was a way of feeling a connection with his dad, and our son. And, there was comfort knowing that in a literal way, my father-in-law lived on in our son.

There were other losses too—not seeing much of family or friends for many months. With the baby blues and being a new mom, I could have used a lot more of that. Our son missed out on socializing and going out a lot that first year of life. Understanding how bad getting COVID could be made those choices easier to make, but it was still frustrating and lonely.

I didn't begin processing how traumatic losing my father-in-law to COVID was until a bit later. It remains one of the worst things my husband and I have experienced. COVID really took so much from us, with the experiences leading up to having our son and after—most of all, losing my father-in-law before his time. But, we continue to take comfort and find joy and strength in our son, and now, our daughter too—another pandemic baby, born in January 2022.

I see my father-in-law when I see my husband driving our son in his Jeep, in my daughter's button nose. We were able to do a celebration of life in September 2021 finally, giving us some closure. We talk more freely about my father-in-law now—what he'd think of our kids, what he'd like to do with them. These days, it's more smiles and laughter than tears and anger.

We persevere. Even where there is pain, even where we can't quite find a reason or meaning—we still find our strength and our joy.

LIZ'S STORY

I've told my story to numerous outlets and was featured in AP News, the *New York Post, Parents Magazine* to name a few. MTV wanted to do a docuseries on my experience, but the thought of worrying about camera equipment in my delivery was the last thing I wanted during that time. *New York Family* and *Westchester Family Magazine* dubbed me as the "Warrior of Westchester," complete with a photo of my post-labor fist raised in the air, baby cradled in the other arm. The image went viral on social media, as this was an iconic symbol of the women enduring the same fears in the early days of the COVID-19 pandemic.

The story I'm sharing here includes details I've never shared because the wounds were too fresh. It's almost an out-of-body experience in hindsight, like a movie, where I look back in hindsight asking myself, "Did that really happen?".

At the end of 2019, just a couple of months before the announcement of a pandemic, I announced I was expecting my second child. Simultaneously, in December of 2019, I fell ill for over a month with a mysterious virus that we would later know as COVID-19. I made numerous trips to urgent care and baffled all the doctors and nurses. They sent me on my way, along with an inhaler and told me to get to the ER if I feel like "I can't breathe." I barely could walk the few blocks home and recall texting my husband: If I'm not home soon, retrace the route to the urgent care center.

I made it home, but ended up in bed for a week, which was challenging with a toddler. As if pregnancy wasn't difficult enough for me, I worked more than I ever had, in anticipation of my unpaid maternity leave as a business owner/freelancer. I wore myself out and was weak from this virus that I feared would hurt my baby (even though doctors assured me that I may be bruising ribs with my cough, but the baby was safe for now).

Then, in January, we heard murmurs of a mysterious virus circulating abroad. While most didn't think much of it, I knew right away this would be a threat. My previous pregnancy occurred during the Zika scares, and I feared the worst. My mama bear instincts made my top priority to protect this unborn child. At the same time, we knew we needed more space with another child on the way. We sold our Brooklyn apartment and set out for the NYC 'burbs—all while I was eight months pregnant.

In February, I almost canceled our movers because I didn't want this virus in my home, but I didn't have much of a choice, carrying an extra nearly fifty pounds on my body, almost ready to pop. We settled safely in our new home, and I still commuted to the city for a couple of weeks for photoshoots, and for a moment this impending threat wasn't on my mind, as I was consumed with nesting in my new oasis and life.

In March, I filmed a segment for Fox 5 on maternity fashion with the owner of the brand Hatch, and the whole crew greeted each other with handshakes with elbows and feet, to avoid the spread of germs "just in case." We all laughed how silly it all was. The next day, we heard on the news that a NYC lawyer near my new home Westchester attended a funeral and bar mitzvah in the same weekend and was patient zero of the pandemic reaching our country.

The next few weeks following that news seemed to be a whirlwind. My NYC friends called me laughing that I just moved to near where the National Guard set up like out of a sci-fi film. I immediately pictured doomsday like *I Am Legend* where they just wiped out the whole area to stop the spread.

My anxiety went through the roof and my body was shaking as I begged my husband to not leave home. He worked in a school in Brooklyn and the teacher's union representative demanded he still went into work daily. He begged his principal to stay home until we knew more, as he had a wife at home that was nine months pregnant and lived fairly close to what was declared the "epicenter of the pandemic." Risking his career, he stayed by my side for the next few days before the entire country went into a forced lockdown.

The next couple of weeks seemed like a dream that wove in and out of a nightmare. I enjoyed being in my little hideaway, away from it all and with my little growing family. At the same time, I documented my experience on social media daily, often in tears and connecting with others sharing this scary experience.

I spent the last couple of weeks of my pregnancy advocating for expecting mothers, who were forced to give birth alone in the initial lockdown period. Giving birth alone is a terrifying through, but at that point it was still unclear about exactly how it was transmitted—if it was airborne or through surfaces, or both. We were still wiping down Amazon boxes and my husband was stripping down and washing his clothes anytime he came home from work before we officially locked down. We didn't know how severe the illness would be, especially for a pregnant person or worse, a newborn child.

At my forty-week appointment with a midwife, I requested a membrane sweep to induce my labor. I wanted the baby safely out of my body and home in my suburban hideout. I think I willed myself to give birth, because the midwife was in disbelief when my contracts immediately were getting closer and closer. By the time I got home they were closer than when they advise to go to the hospital. My husband urged me to get my hospital bag, but I didn't want to spend more time in the hospital than was necessary.

Despite unwarranted advice on social media, I also knew I didn't want a home birth. Not only was it impossible to get someone to come to your home, I knew that my mom had a complicated birth and being in a hospital saved my life in my last birth. Either way, giving birth in the early peak of the pandemic was a risky situation.

Down to the wire, we raced to the hospital that seemed like an eternity away. With limited staff, there was no valet and seemingly no parking spaces. We were circling the parking lot of White Plains Hospital with contractions coming two minutes apart. I was afraid if I went into the building without my husband while he parked the car, he might not be allowed in.

They were extremely strict on partners at the time and the new mandate was to allow one person in for the birth pending they tested negative for the virus, wore a mask, and left following the birth. I felt for all the women that had to go through it alone, as they still weren't allowing partners in the hospital just days prior to my birth, but luckily the governor ruled that to be inhumane.

One of the hospital staff noticed that I was doubled over with contractions in the parking lot and wheeled a wheelchair over to scoop me up. They stopped my husband and did numerous tests and questioned him, while they brought me straight to the delivery room. I soaked through the surgical mask they gave me while I was in tears between the contractions and worries that they wouldn't let my husband in. We reunited not too long after and they gave me a fresh mask.

An hour later, our test results came in virus-free, so the staff stripped down their PPE gear, which could only be compared to when ET was being observed by medical staff. The entire room relaxed, and as did I. Though, I still requested an epidural because between wearing a mask and the anxiety, it wasn't helping me progress in my labor. I hardly remember the pain of the shot in my spine, but I'll never forget that only the right half of my body went numb, which was almost laughable with everything going on.

Having a doula virtually also helped guide me through the process, as this birth was a stark contrast to my first birth experience. I felt so fortunate that under the circumstances of a short-staffed and overwhelmed hospital, I at least went in knowing what to expect.

Still, when I told the nurse that I was ready to push, she replied, "You're going to have to wait." If you've ever delivered a baby naturally (especially a second child) you know there's no "waiting." My doula knew from being with me for now two births, it was time and on FaceTime, insisted that the nurse called the doctor. Sure enough, the doctor entered the room, took one look and said, "Good thing she got me. That baby wants out and you're ready to push!" I hadn't even met any of the ob-gyns because they were all called into the hospitals full-time. I had only been with the medical practice for a month prior and only saw PAs and midwives. I first met the OB that delivered my baby right as she delivered the baby!

It was a huge relief that she was here safely with me, but the biggest fears were to come. The mandate at the time was for husbands/partners to only be present for the birth but would have to return home for the mother's recovery. In my previous birth, I hemorrhaged so much that my OB had to give me something to stop it and put me under observation. I was worried that if I passed out and there was no one in the room to advocate for me, then I could bleed to death. This happened to someone in a documentary I watched on the Black Maternal Health Crisis—and she was ignored. I feared I was to be ignored, for other reasons of course. I begged to be observed for this and for my husband to stay just a little longer. They obliged and kept my bleeding under control.

I gave birth at 5:30 p.m. and promptly at 7 p.m. they sent me off to recovery and told my husband to go home—for the best night of sleep he's had in years! I, on the other hand, experienced fear, and neglect for the next day or so. I asked for Motrin to get ahead of the pain and didn't receive it for over twenty hours because the pharmacy was so backed up. I asked when I would receive dinner after not eating all day and birthing a human, but the staff replied that the kitchen was closed. Luckily a kind nurse took pity on me and found a pint of salad that was mostly iceberg lettuce, but at least some nourishment. I noshed on my homemade lactation balls, which was the only sustenance for both me and my breastfed baby for the next twelve hours or so following the birth.

I asked a nurse to help me to the bathroom because I was in so much pain and couldn't move. She offered me a bedpan, from a distance in fear herself of getting sick without my mask on for a moment. I crawled on the floor to the toilet while she stood there and watched me wipe down and cover the seat, worried about the germs. I even refused to even shower, worried about leaving my baby alone (not to mention in fear of catching the virus).

All I wanted to do was go home and get my baby out of there. They kept us longer than I hoped because they had to do extra testing on her (which turned out to be nothing) and I sat in my room alone, shaking, every time they'd wheel her bassinet out to the nursery to poke and prod her. After thirty hours I was released back home to begin the postpartum journey in lockdown, which while I was relieved to be home safely with my baby, it seemed the fears didn't go away. I worried about her safety every minute, as we had no idea what the virus's effects on infants, let alone a newborn, could be. To add to my worries, what kind of world I brought her into. I was terrified if I would have a career in styling now that my industry shut down. I was scared for my toddler, not fully aware of what was happening, but aware enough that he started to get anxiety from our fears.

Postpartum during COVID-19 had negatives for sure, but it was magical to have that time with just our family and no one else. It forced me to be fully present with my kids, which I may never have again. I'm also so grateful that I was able to connect virtually with so many other women going through this experience at the same time.

My doula once said at my first birth that lasted over twenty-four hours that she would power through because "I'm a warrior!!" Now I always say after this birth experience during a pandemic, we are truly warrior mamas. Our babies are warriors too. My little girl (named after my late mother's nickname, which also aptly means "courage") is the most strong-willed and confident little girl I've ever met and I think my pandemic baby gave me that courage.

CLARK'S STORY

I found out I was pregnant with my second son exactly a month before the State of Louisiana, which is where I was located at the time, shut down. When I had found out I was pregnant, I was really excited, obviously, because we were going to have another baby and I was excited to have what I was calling a "normal" pregnancy. My first son was born in Hawaii, and we were thousands of miles away from close friends and family. We had a few friends on island, but I didn't have the support of the people that I really wanted to have around me when I was expecting my first baby. I also didn't get to have certain experiences you come to expect with pregnancy. I didn't have a baby shower with my close friends or family, and they weren't at the delivery. My family mailed me maternity clothes because there weren't maternity clothes to buy on island. I remember saying to my husband when we found out we were pregnant with our second child, that I was really excited to be able to get a proper bra fitting for being pregnant and go to some maternity or prenatal yoga classes and connect with other pregnant women.

We had planned that we were going to get to tell our family in person that we were expecting because they were supposed to visit us within the next couple months. It felt like we were going to get the opportunity that we did not get to have when we lived in Hawaii. To then find out a month later, everything was shutting down, was hard. I hadn't even gotten in to see an OB at that point to confirm my pregnancy in person. With the shutdown, obviously didn't know exactly what that meant, but it was definitely a feeling of uncertainty throughout the course of my pregnancy. With the implementation of stay-at-home orders and social distancing, all our plans, and more, became dreams rather than anticipated realities.

Throughout my entire pregnancy, my husband was only able to come to one appointment. Whereas in our first pregnancy, he came to almost every single appointment, he may have missed one. Although, I do think I had the advantage that this was not my first pregnancy. I didn't feel as nervous going to certain doctor's appointments as I had the first time, but I would've liked for him to have been there and to be able to see the ultrasound and to be able to see those things was something we had not expected.

What was probably the hardest for me during the pregnancy during COVID was the isolation and feeling alone. I also felt exhausted because day care was shut down, so my oldest son was home with us too. Trying to balance being pregnant, taking care of my son and working, along with managing all the anxieties and fears and worries that came with the pandemic, was a lot.

I was really looking forward to that pregnancy, being able to be surrounded by close friends that I had locally in Louisiana and get to celebrate the pregnancy with them, but we couldn't do that. We were able to have a gender reveal with just a few friends, but we social distanced. It was just a few friends because again, we didn't want to be with large groups and with the regulations regarding gathering size at the time, I don't even think we could gather in large groups then. We were able to share the gender reveal over Zoom with family and friends elsewhere, but it just didn't quite feel the same.

I definitely think my anxiety intensified in the pregnancy because of the anxiety of COVID—with it not safe to be around people and having to isolate. In preparing for the birth of my second son, we had to have conversations with my doctor and family to prepare, because as part of our life as a military family our family was still not close to us. While we were back in the continental US, my family was in Pennsylvania and my husband's family was in Virginia. We had to take a lot of precautions because of the pandemic. After talking to our doctors, we decided we had to have our family isolate two weeks prior to them coming to visit; they drove instead of flying and they had to isolate on the trip down to us. We had to ask a lot of them, and we had to do a lot. My doctor had recommended that my husband, son, and I quarantine for two weeks before the delivery so there was less risk of contracting COVID. If we did contract COVID, there could be the issue of having to be separated from the baby because I believe at that time, they were still isolating moms from babies if the mom was positive for COVID. So, two weeks before delivery, my husband wasn't able to go to work and my son (who we had sent back to preschool that fall) had to come home for two weeks and stay home for a few weeks after the birth too.

About a week before I was scheduled for my C-section my husband just started to have a little bit of a stuffy nose and out of abundance of precaution we wanted to get tested. He went to get a test (this was in

October of 2020) and there were so many different tests that were out there. Some were much more reliable than others. My husband called me while he was still at the testing site, and he said it came back positive. Immediately my reaction was, "There's no way. There's no way that your test came back positive for COVID. There's no way, can you ask them to test you again?" And he told me they said, "No, it's positive. You're positive."

He came home and they told us he had to immediately isolate, which meant I was thirty-eight, thirty-nine weeks pregnant and had to do everything around the household, including care for my husband and care for my two-year-old. All while I was very, very pregnant. At the time I told him, I really thought he should get another test because I just didn't feel like it was accurate, especially since his test results said that test was 88 percent reliable. There's a big difference between that and 98 percent reliability. In the meantime, I had reached out to my doctor's office at the time, and I told them what happened and explained I didn't think that my husband was actually positive for COVID because he didn't have a fever, he barely had a stuffy nose, we'd not been around anybody, and he was going to get another test. My doctor's office called me back and we were told that my husband could no longer come with me to the delivery. It felt like my world stopped. I completely broke down. There was so little that I had control over in my life at that time because so many things were dictated by pregnancy or COVID. This was the one thing that we were expecting—that my husband was going to be there. We took all the precautions, we did all the right things, and I was just devastated. I was in hysterics.

The next COVID test that my husband took did come back negative, but when I called the doctor and let them know that they still said he could not come. So, we decided to get my husband a third test. In the midst of this, I called my parents in hysterics and said, "How soon can you get down here?" They were planning to drive to our house in a few days, right before the scheduled C-section to watch our oldest son, but now if I went into labor before they got there, we didn't have anybody that could watch my son, with my husband, having tested positive. I also needed somebody to get there because I wasn't ready to have the baby yet. The house still wasn't together, my bag wasn't fully packed, and I not only needed help with my son, but I needed someone to come to the hospital with me. It was a two-day drive for my parents to get to our house. They were able to move their schedule around a little to make it a day earlier.

My mom was going to come for the delivery with me. I was just beside myself. I remember over the course of those few days that I was so stressed and was having some contractions I think because of the stress of having to do everything for myself, my husband, and my son. It was completely wearing on me. Also, it was just really upsetting to think that we had taken all the precautions, we did all the right things, we followed all the guidelines and that he wasn't going to get to be at the delivery.

My husband got a third test. This was during the time when there wasn't rapid testing, so it would take like a couple days to get the results back. Once we got the results and were able to call my doctor with two negative test results, they said they were going to assume that the first test was false. So, they finally agreed that my husband could come to the delivery, just a couple days before I was scheduled for my C-section. My parents were still able to get to our house a little earlier, but emotionally it was a lot leading up to that.

We had a great delivery, and we had a great experience at the hospital. I think I experienced postpartum anxiety after my first son, and I knew what to look for. So, I think that was good. My anxiety definitely revved up a lot in postpartum with my second son for several reasons. We were discharged home two hours before Hurricane Zeta hit New Orleans (which is where we were living). Two hours after we arrived home, we lost power for three days. My husband and I ended up having to go to a hotel for a few days because I had just given birth and couldn't be without power. I needed to get sleep, to be able to shower and to have running water for me and this brand-new baby. At the same time, we had to constantly weigh the risks of exposing ourselves and exposing this brand-new baby to COVID and germs, so it was stressful.

For probably six months after my son was born it was really intense for me. I couldn't have people necessarily come over. We experienced so much isolation. There was the constant risk-benefit analysis. "I need to go to this doctor's appointment, or I need to take the baby to this place, but like, what if I expose him? Does the risk outweigh the benefit?" It was really, really stressful and really, really isolating.

About a month or two after my second son was born, I was having a rough day with my oldest son. My friend came over to help, but because of concern about the risks of exposure she couldn't really hold the baby. We also couldn't hire a babysitter that could stay with the baby so I could go back to work. Once my son was three or four months old, we were just at the beginning stage of vaccinations, so that started to bring some hope.

I am very grateful that this experience did not happen with my first baby. I did feel like I was robbed of a lot of things that I was really looking forward to, but I had gotten to experience what a more normal (than being in COVID) pregnancy and delivery looked like.

Interestingly enough, I recently found out I am pregnant with our third child and am holding my breath. I'm not going to say it's going to be normal, but I feel it is going to be different in many capacities than the last one. My husband was already able to come to the first doctor's appointment, which couldn't even happen before. We will see how this all plays out.

Pregnancy is typically a time filled with celebration, joy, and eager expectation of your little one's arrival. During pregnancy, there are milestones you look forward to: the first time you hear your baby's heartbeat, seeing that tiny little face on an ultrasound, a gender reveal party, a baby shower thrown by loved ones, and the first time you get to finally hold your bundle of joy in your arms. Throughout those special moments, you can't wait to share them with your partner or spouse, other children, friends, and family members. With the arrival of the pandemic, those of us who were pregnant found that our expectations for many of those milestones seemed to shatter around us.

I think being pregnant during COVID-19 was something that, if you went through it, you understand what that felt like. And it's hard to explain to someone who wasn't pregnant or had a baby during that time. The level of isolation and uncertainty. I just hope that we never have to go through something like that again. Knowing that we did get through it, it's hard, but hopefully it's not something that continues to impact us in a traumatic way.

ALESSANDRA'S STORY

I remember asking my midwife if coronavirus was something I needed to be worried about, as she checked the heartbeat of my third baby. I was thankful my older two children were there to witness that sound for the first time, but never did it occur to me, it would also be the last time.

She was honest with me and said I needed to be careful but there really wasn't anything she knew that I didn't know. So, I walked out of the appointment with my kids and a positive attitude. I thought to myself, I don't get sick often anyway, so I probably don't have to worry too much.

I announced my pregnancy later that day "officially" on social media. I was about fourteen weeks along. One week later the world shut down.

I spent the remainder of my pregnancy going to appointments alone or having them over the phone. I remember thinking how unfair it was to have a telehealth appointment while pregnant. The whole point of those appointments was to make sure my baby's heartbeat was still there. And as someone who had suffered miscarriage, this was even more grueling.

My husband was unable to attend appointments, as well. Missing out on all those "lasts" because we knew this would be our final baby. The halfway scan, the glucose test, the nonstress test at the very end, all done alone. I guess in reality it was going to happen anyway as my husband would have either stayed home with our older kids or would have been working, but the mere fact that he couldn't be there was what hurt. I felt bad he missed it all.

But I also know I was lucky to have him by my side during labor. Like so many pregnant women, I was fearful I would have to deliver alone after hearing so many stories of other women going alone. It brings tears to my eyes just thinking about those brave moms!

Once it was "go time" my husband and I headed to the hospital for our last baby's birth, with hospital bags and masks in hand. I will never forget or get over the fact that I needed to labor and deliver my baby with a mask on my face! It actually wasn't as bad as it sounds, I think I was a little preoccupied with other things, but it's still crazy to think about. When I had my six-week postpartum appointment, my midwife didn't even recognize me. She asked how my delivery went and I said, "Well you delivered my baby!" She felt terrible of course, and we know it was because of the masks. She had never even seen my face, and vice versa!

But that wasn't even the worst part. I hated that my two older children weren't allowed to visit us in the hospital. That was a moment I was so excited about at the beginning of my pregnancy that was taken from me. We waited to find out until delivery if we were having a boy or girl, and my older kids had to learn over a FaceTime call.

The question I get asked the most though is, "What was the transition to three kids like?" People automatically think it was my hardest transition, but honestly it was the easiest. And I truly think I have COVID to thank for that.

I may have missed out on mom groups, had to go to doctor appointments alone, and had telehealth midwife visits, too. But I gained so much more. Who would have ever thought something good could come from this?

But COVID allowed for slower days at home. Less activities and events where I had to get three kids ready or cart them all around on my own. And even though my kids were able to go back to school in the fall of 2020, the biggest blessing in disguise was …

My husband was working from home through it all. Not having to be alone at home while transitioning from two to three kids was everything. My husband was home so I could bring my infant to her doctor appointments without getting all three kids in the car. When I had to do school pickup and the baby was sleeping, she was able to stay home and sleep. I had constant support from the person who meant the most.

My husband got to watch firsthand what it was truly like for me to be a stay-at-home mom and a new appreciation was felt through that. He got to stay home with his third child too! I watched him appreciate the newborn phase so much more and grow and bond with our third baby more than he was able to with our first two babies because he had time.

Going through postpartum during COVID was honestly the best postpartum experience I've had. It allowed me the support I would not have had before, and that every single mom deserves.

I think this should be a lesson for so many of us, that a husband's/spouse's support through postpartum (that's longer than two weeks!) is so, so important for moms and babies. Not only do new mothers need and deserve that constant support, but our husbands deserve that time, too.

COVID gave us all moments we will never forget, both good and bad. But mostly, it gave us memories, family support, and time. And we learned that there's always a silver lining to be found, even in the darkest of times.

JULIE'S STORY

My son Rafi was born on March 14, 2020, at exactly thirty-seven weeks' gestation. Given that the Louisiana governor shut things down on March 13, 2020, Rafi was one of the first babies to be born into the early pandemic world. Between 2016 and 2020, my husband and I experienced a never-ending rollercoaster of highs and lows as we struggled with infertility. Rafi and his older brother by two and a half years, Gabe, were both IVF miracle babies. My pregnancy with Gabe ended at thirty-two-and-a-half weeks, and I had several miscarriages in between the births of my sons. We were so happy to be completing our family with miracle baby number two, and we were so looking forward to a normal, nontraumatic birthing experience ... we were totally unprepared for what was about to happen!

In order to (hopefully) keep Rafi in utero until at least thirty-seven weeks, I had weekly progesterone shots for most of the pregnancy. Those shots left my upper arm throbbing for several minutes after each injection, but they were a tiny price to pay to stay free of the NICU this time around. Although I was thirty-eight with a toddler that I was not supposed to lift and at high risk for age and diabetes (not gestational), it was a fairly easy pregnancy. COVID-19 was only in the back of our minds because my husband's family lives in Italy and we were concerned that the virus affecting Asia and Europe would prevent them from coming to New Orleans shortly after Rafi's birth. We took zero precautions. We even did a little bit of Mardi Gras parading two and a half weeks before the shutdown. As an aside, Mardi Gras 2020 turned out to be a super-spreader event leaving New Orleans as one of the major hotspots early on. I was uncomfortable being pregnant, but my family was fine and definitely had no clue what was coming next. My focus was on staying pregnant so we wouldn't have another traumatic birthing experience and a long NICU stay.

My older son was born seven and a half weeks before his due date. I had woken up early in excruciating pain on the last day of August 2017, and since I had never been in labor before and more so that my baby was not due until late October, being in full-blown labor was the last thing on my mind. After an hour or so wishing the pain away, my husband drove me to the hospital. Gabe was breach, so the medical team said we need to do an emergency C-section. A few hours later, I became Mommy to a three-pound, fourteen-ounce beautiful blonde-haired, blue-eyed baby boy. I was told to expect a long NICU stay, because most preterm babies are not ready to go home until their due date. NICU days spent trying to pump breast milk were long, scary, and frustrating, but Gabriel (Hebrew for God is my strength) was a fighter, and he broke out of that NICU exactly five weeks later, at *thirty-seven and a half weeks'* gestation. Since Gabe was so tiny and flu season was upon us, we were regularly advised to keep him away from the public for as long as possible. At four months old, even though we were fearful to remove Gabe's shield, we ripped off the band aid and sent him to school.

Fast forward to March 13, 2020. I was thirty-six weeks and six days and so uncomfortable that I was ready for Rafi to join our family. Governor Edwards held a press conference midday and announced that schools were closing for two weeks. I was stressed because that meant Gabe would have a long, early spring break. My back started hurting throughout the day and by 7 p.m. that night I said, "We need to go to the hospital." The discomfort felt similar to going into labor at thirty-two-and-a-half weeks, so I didn't want to take any chances. The doctor checked me and told me I was not dilated at all yet, that they were giving me some pain meds and sending me home. I was disappointed because I was ready to be DONE. Then the nurse took my blood pressure, and it was 200+/80 (I hadn't had any BP problems prior) and I was told I was not going home, but instead due to my newly discovered preeclampsia, I was having this baby tonight.

I needed a C-section and I had eaten something a few hours before, so I had to wait until the next morning before they could operate. Rafi arrived the next morning and he was healthy enough to stay in the room with me. Although my experience was anything but normal, at least Rafi, my husband, and I were together. The hospital was a ghost town. No visitors allowed. Protocols were rapidly changing, staffing was limited, and everyone was scared. My husband could come and go the first few days so he could see Gabe who was staying with my parents, but pretty quickly he was not allowed to leave not only the hospital, but the actual maternity floor, if he wanted to get back in. The hospital was completely unprepared. I avoided the news because I was avoiding this new world that we would leave the hospital as long as I could.

The morning after Rafi was born, I was anxious to finally get out of bed.

That would be delayed, however, as I started gushing blood. I remember the nurses weighing my soaked sheets as they scrambled to figure out what was going on. I remember feeling so cold and like I was dying, but I did not want to be separated from my baby. They took me to the pre-op area and gave me two units of blood. I started feeling better. If that had not worked, they were going to take me back into surgery. It would have been nice to have had my mom around during this unwanted adventure.

And when we thought things could not get any more stressful, Rafi became very jaundiced and spent the next five days under the blue light. They kept pricking his tiny feet to squeeze blood out and it was terribly heart-wrenching especially without family support. When we finally were discharged, at what was identical to Gabe's discharge at *thirty-seven and a half weeks'* gestation, the entrance to the hospital felt like a war zone with masked nurses doing temperature checks. During the twenty-minute drive home, it was like we were in a hopeless, abandoned world.

We brought our new baby home to finally meet his grandparents and big brother and the six of us became a "pod," always together for the next several months. Once we were home, the only help we had was from my parents. It was eerily similar to bringing Gabe home, but in retrospect, it was so much worse. Friends would come by and stand in front our big window to get a glimpse of our new addition. Nobody could meet Rafi. It was very isolating and surreal.

The challenges seemed like they would never be complete. The many new baby pediatrician and specialist appointments with just one parent allowed in the room were awful. All the protocols of masks and temperature checks and isolation were excruciating. There was so much fear of the unknown! So much information and misinformation was flowing in and none of us knew what was coming next. The constant fear of getting COVID—who would live and who would die? This was exacerbated for me because of all the post-baby hormones! There was no real maternity leave because I had my two-and-a-half-year-old and my newborn home together for five and a half straight months, binging *Cocomelon*, until we nervously put them in school. As anxiety-provoking as it was, we had to do it though. We had to work, and the boys, especially Gabe, needed socialization.

No, I did not get the normal childbirth experience with Rafi that I so longed for. I did get a new perspective, however. Rafi's name Raphael (Hebrew for God has healed) was chosen before the pandemic because he was a last-chance IVF miracle and thus healing for our souls. We could never have imagined that our child Raphael would be our healer for the "pandemic world" as well. He was the ship that kept us afloat for nearly two years of rough COVID waters.

Our buzzword of 2020/2021 was fluid. The experiences the boys had at school parallel to the experiences we were witnessing at work, were uncomfortably too fluid, giving new meaning to go with the flow. But we did it, and we came out OK on the other side. My takeaway for new moms in a future crisis—don't give up, hold your kid(s) tight, and try to enjoy every milestone, even if the world around you is dark and seems to be falling apart, because our babies grow so fast. Hang in there. It will get better, I promise.

ALLISON'S STORY

I gave birth to my son in May 2020 at Sibley Hospital in Washington, DC. When everything shut down, I was, for the most part, able to feel optimistic and relatively content about how things were going with my pregnancy and about the silver linings that the pandemic did afford; I didn't have to commute for the last two months of my pregnancy, I was able to wear sweatpants and slippers while working, and I enjoyed being home. But the scariest part was the concern about whether my husband would be able to be in the room with me during the birth. I followed the news with trepidation as we heard that New York hospitals had banned partners from attending their children's births in March. I then felt some relief upon hearing that the governor of New York had overturned that ban, but still certainly held some anxiety of the unknown. The doctor who saw me for my thirty-seven-week appointment was the one who informed me that the hospital where I would deliver was beginning to test the birthing parents, and if the birthing parent tested positive for COVID, the other parent would not be able to stay. That happened to be the same doctor who was on call when I was in labor, and I remember saying to my doula (on Zoom of course …) that I didn't like this doctor. I assume that at my most vulnerable, I felt this dislike because of my association with her as the deliverer of a scary possibility.

We interviewed our doula on March 12, 2020, and she happened to mention that if hospitals stopped allowing further in-person visitors, she had experience with virtual support. By the time we made our decision about who to hire a couple weeks later, that was certainly the component of her experience that stood out and felt most relevant to our choice. On March 20, I had my thirty-two-week appointment, at which the ob-gyn office gave me a survey to screen for postpartum depression. The survey asked questions such as: "Have you felt more anxious this week?" or

21

"Have you cried more this week?" I felt like my answers to both questions were yes, but I also knew that this was because of the world shutting down and not because of pregnancy and hormones. While I understand the vital importance of doing one's best to screen for genuine depression, it felt almost comical to try to answer these questions during that week.

Despite everything, my birth experience itself was quite positive: I had two goals, but I knew it was better to be pleasantly surprised if they were accomplished rather than disappointed if they didn't happen. But both happened as I wanted! We chose not to find out the sex of our baby, and our doula asked my husband if he wanted to announce the sex to me. He was able to do so and it's a wonderful and special memory that I will relish forever. The other achievement is that despite having a doula on Zoom, I was able to give birth naturally without an epidural, which I was also very proud of, and our doula and her team were especially impressed with as well. Of course, some aspects of the birth experience in the hospital were different than they otherwise would have been: The nursery was closed, the waiting rooms were closed, no visitors were allowed, and my husband had to stay the whole time. He could not leave and return for any reason once we were there. The delivering doctor wore a face shield, and I was supposed to wear a mask but once my test came back negative, they were not very particular about that.

Ironically, many parts of our hospital stay felt the most normal and removed from the pandemic than either my husband or I had felt in months. A nurse was chatting with me at approximately 3 a.m. on the second night and apologized to me for being so chatty. I could not emphasize to her enough the degree to which she did not need to apologize! I had a thirty-six-hour-old baby who could not be in the nursery because it was closed, so despite my husband's best efforts, I was not sleeping at all, and hers was the first regular, chitchat conversation I had had with someone I did not know in over two months. I was so grateful for the small talk at three in the morning.

I find that in retrospect, it can sometimes be easy to think about how we should have done things differently and forget how little we knew in the moment. In those first weeks at the end of March, we held out hope that lockdowns and restrictions would last only a couple weeks, and that we would be able to celebrate our child in person with our friends, family, and community. Only as my due date drew closer did we realize that would not be the case. As a Jewish family, we planned to have a welcome and naming ceremony for our child on the eighth day of their life, which would include a bris (circumcision) if he was a boy. My husband and I have large extended families who reliably show up to family events, and as it happened, the eighth day of our son's life was on the Sunday of Memorial Day weekend. Had his birth happened under any other circumstances, we would have had a large, celebratory gathering to mark this occasion. Instead, my husband, son, and I were joined in our home only by the person performing the circumcision, known as the mohel. When the mohel came inside, masked, it was the first time anyone besides us had been inside our house in two months, and it felt very notable. Although we had 150 people from all over the world attend the ceremony via Zoom, we still grieve the missed experience of having an in-person gathering when our son was eight days old.

Because of this, in 2023, we planned a big third birthday party for our son with lots of family invited from out of town, because we were very eager to celebrate him with family and friends in person in a way that we were not able to when he was born. We hope to someday also have a second child and are optimistic that those aspects of the experience will be very different the second time around. We are grateful that our son will not remember the experience of 2020, but we know that he will certainly learn about it as an integral part of the story of how he came into the world.

ERICA'S STORY

I entered my third trimester right when the COVID lockdown hit. One of the hardest things about the end of my pregnancy was that I couldn't really share it with anyone. We had canceled my baby shower, and I didn't realize how much I needed and wanted that rite of passage until I didn't have it. My belly wasn't super noticeable until that third trimester, and it sounds so silly, but I wanted to have the experience of someone giving up their seat for me on the metro or have some stranger ask to put their hand on my belly. Instead, I just sort of disappeared from the world, like some Victorian woman who had to enter her period of "confinement." When I reemerged, I felt like no one (aside from my husband) had witnessed this huge physical and emotional change I had experienced.

By the time I went into labor in June 2020, the rules around COVID had become more predictable. I could have my husband with me at the hospital, but not anyone else. And we had to wear masks.

The masks contributed to some of the more memorable moments of my birth experience. As a first-time mom, I had assumed my labor would progress slowly, so I wanted to labor at home as long as possible. Well, I waited too long. My contractions were three to four minutes apart (instead of the recommended five to seven minutes), by the time I waddled out to the car to drive to the hospital. Just as we reached the end of our block, we realized that we had forgotten to pack our masks. There were still mask shortages at this point, including in health care settings, so we turned the car around. My husband dashed inside our home, grabbed the masks, and dashed out again, terrified that the baby would come before we managed the twenty-minute drive to the hospital in downtown Washington, D.C.

Thankfully, we made it in time. My labor continued to progress quite rapidly, and the second mask-related moment happened while I was still in triage, with just a flimsy curtain separating me from the woman in the next bed. As I entered the transition phase of labor—that really painful phase right before you're ready to push—the pain made me so nauseous that I threw up. (It turns out, there's a reason they say not to eat a full meal after you start active labor!) Only, I didn't manage to get my mask off fast enough, so I just ended up projectile vomiting into my mask. The whole thing is hilarious now, but, at that moment, I remember thinking that I needed to try to somehow salvage my now compromised mask. My husband, who was thinking more clearly in that moment, stepped in and just threw it away, and the nurse provided me with a clean mask, just in time for delivery.

Giving birth was one of the most empowering experiences of my life. Because of how quickly my labor progressed, I was able to do the natural birth that I had hoped for. The fact that I pushed a human out of me, while wearing a mask, continues to make me feel like a badass. :-) In fact, by the time it came to push, I didn't even register that I had a mask on.

There were a lot of mixed emotions to becoming a mom and bringing a baby into the world during a global pandemic. On the positive side, my husband and I were both at home and had a lot of time together with our son, especially in those early months of his life. We got to celebrate his "firsts" in an incredibly intimate way. And his growth and development marked the passage of time, giving us hope and meaning at a time when COVID made much of life seem meaningless.

But there was also a lot of grief at the things we missed out on. I had wanted to be a "cool mom," someone who continued to meet up with friends, passed the baby around a lot, and went about my regular life, just with a baby strapped on in a carrier. Instead, I just went on a lot of stroller walks by myself. My best friend didn't hold my son until he was a year old, and my grandmother only met him once before she passed away. Writing in my journal a few months after my son was born, I summed up these experiences with Dickens: "It was the best of times; it was the worst of times."

ASHLEY'S STORY

At the very beginning of March, my husband and I found out we were pregnant. At the end of March, we were going to be traveling from Kansas City to Florida for my mother-in-law's sixtieth birthday—to surprise her. We were also going to surprise our whole family and tell them the news!

We had traveled in February when stories about COVID were just beginning to surface, and it was still being compared to the flu. When things started to get more serious by mid-March and there was talk about shutting everything down, we started to get worried that maybe travel wasn't the best idea. We didn't know what could happen as there weren't a lot of details about how this could affect a mother or a baby—so we had to tell our family why we were nervous and our big surprise was less big because it had to happen over FaceTime.

My husband and I both worked in jobs that had us in people's houses every day and as a personal chef, he was in and out of the grocery store twice a day every day. We were worried about what he could bring home, I mean at that point there was no real solid information. We both stayed home, and he would drive me to doctors' appointments, but not be allowed to come in. I heard the heartbeat by myself. The very first baby I would ever have, and I got my first sonogram alone. I watched the baby wiggle around alone, and I heard his heartbeat with the sonogram tech. I took a video, and we watched in the car together while we waited for AAA because my husband's car battery died while he was waiting for me—HA!

The very first sonogram my husband got to see for that baby was at the end of May after a night of debilitating pain brought us to the emergency room. We had called the after-hours line twice that night and were told to come into the office first thing in the morning so they could do a sonogram and that with everything going on they didn't want to send me to the ER. At 5–6 a.m. I just couldn't take what I later learned were contractions

26

anymore, and we left for the hospital. My husband called ahead to determine if he was even going to be allowed to come in.

Once we got checked in, they called me in and as soon as I walked through the door, I felt the blood. Doctors and nurses were coming in and getting vitals and asking lots of questions—and finally, the sonogram tech came in. He wouldn't show us the screen or really talk to us at all, and it wasn't until the emergency room doctor came in to confirm that we had lost our boy that we knew it was over.

I will never forget that doctor's eyes because that's all I could see, and they said everything. It was a whirlwind morning and I had to go into surgery. The doctor literally said the baby wasn't where he should be and I made the tech show me again himself. I had been laboring and didn't know, at fourteen weeks.

I woke up in recovery by myself because no one was allowed to be back in recovery. I didn't remember why I was there, and I looked at the nurse and asked and she told me. I just remember the bottom falling out and crying and not having anyone there to talk to about it.

As I gathered myself up to leave and changed back into clothes, the nurse offered me the big water bottle and I politely declined letting her know that I didn't want any souvenirs from the day. She wheeled me out to the curb and I got in my husband's car and we left …

All things considered, the doctors, nurses, and all the staff we interacted with that day couldn't have been nicer and really made the experience less awful than I guess it could've been. What do you do after a loss like that in the middle of a pandemic? We just went back to work … and, life.

I was pregnant again in March 2021 a year later when things were more "open" but still very much locked down. My husband was allowed at appointments, but we had to be masked and I didn't see my doctor's face until July 2023 for the first time! What a time to be alive!

Now—in August of 2023 we have a twenty-one-month-old rainbow baby who is amazing, wonderful, and special. It's hard to grieve your loss when you are looking at this wonderful boy and know that he wouldn't exist this way if what happened before hadn't happened. It's hard to be almost thirty-six with only one child imagining that you could be done with kids by now … and they could be closer in age. Therapy has taught me that the pain will never go away and that a loss like we experienced is just hard. I wouldn't wish it on anyone.

J'S STORY

I was due April 19, 2020, but due to a prior fibroid surgery my MFM determined that I needed to have a C-section three weeks early, to avoid the risk of uterine rupture. As March approached and things in NYC began to shut down, hospitals started to say that partners would not be allowed at births. Other pregnant women started to research going out of state so that their husbands/partners could be with them, but for me that was not an option because of my complicated situation. Luckily for us, right before the date of our scheduled C-section, NY Presbyterian determined that partners could be present for the delivery portion of the birth.

On March 30, 2020, my husband and I went to Weill Cornell Medical Center, and I was given an old-school COVID test, where it felt like they were trying to reach for my brain, and it hurt so badly it made me cry. I was then prepared for my C-section, and then pretty quickly thereafter, our son was born. After a short while we were brought into a recovery area and my husband was permitted to hold our son for a few minutes, and then he was told he would have to leave the hospital, and he could not come back until it was time to pick us up at the end of our stay. We were very upset to have to say goodbye but there was nothing we could do about it, and we were glad that he was able to be there for at least a couple hours.

We were taken to a private room which was actually really nice, so I was excited! I was informed this was just because the results of my COVID test had not come back yet, and I would be in the private room just until the results came back. The first night was rough. Friends had told me not to be shy about sending the baby to the nursery to get some sleep. Well, there was no nursery, it was closed for COVID. Moreover, there was no husband because he had been sent home. Whenever I called the nurses, they rarely if ever came. I got behind on my pain meds because the nurses wouldn't show up on time with the meds. I would page them, and they just wouldn't

28

show up. I would ask for help with diaper changes or breastfeeding and they would tell me I needed to figure it out on my own. But figuring it out on my own, when I still had a catheter in, and had a deep, painful incision through my abdomen, was really not that easy to do. I ended up giving our son formula when he was screaming because I couldn't figure out breastfeeding and the lactation consultants just wouldn't show up, and I just didn't know what else to do. Not that there is anything wrong with formula, but in hindsight, the total lack of support I received at the beginning of my breastfeeding journey with my son probably doomed it from the start.

The next morning, I woke up and they told me it was time to take out the catheter. So, they took out the catheter and then I went to use the bathroom in the hospital room. While I was in there, someone came and started taking all of my things! My baby was lying there in the bassinet, being pushed around by all of the hubbub and I freaked out and started screaming when I saw what was going on. The man who was grabbing my luggage said that he had been given an order to move my things to another room. I ran out into the hall to get a nurse to ask what was going on. She said that my COVID test came back negative, so I was being moved to a double. I told her that was fine, but this was not an appropriate way to do this, I would have liked to have been told, and not to have my stuff moved while I was in the bathroom, and my baby was in the room all alone without me.

As it turns out, I was moved into a room with a woman I knew. We had met years ago through a common friend. It was really nice to see a common face. She had just had her second C-section and was able to tell me how different this experience was from when she had her first child several years prior. While it all seemed crazy to me, hearing it from someone who had a comparison point was grounding. At one point I overheard my friend ask for tea, so then I asked for tea as well. The nurse looked at me and said, "If you want tea, go out in the hallway and get yourself tea." I looked at her kind of surprised and said, "I thought we were really not supposed to be roaming the hallways, and plus, I didn't think we were supposed to leave our babies alone?" The nurse said, "Well if you want tea, go and get it. The babies are on rollers, you can take him with you." There was clearly no chance I was taking a day-old baby into the hallway in the hospital in the middle of a pandemic, but I was shocked at the nurse's callous attitude towards me. It was basically like that my entire stay there.

We had booked a baby nurse to come and stay at our apartment for six weeks and essentially teach us how to parent. The baby nurse came with lots of recommendations and a hefty price tag, but we were sure it would be worth it, as we knew we would want to be able to get some sleep in those first weeks. We had also invested in some of the bougier baby items like the SNOO and the Nanit. So basically, we thought we had the baby game all figured out, we just hadn't planned on a pandemic coming in to wreak havoc on these plans. The baby nurse called me while I was still in the hospital (day two) and said that she would need to cancel, because "in case I hadn't noticed, there was a pandemic out there." No way. Impossible. We had a deal! She said that she was extremely concerned that she would come stay with us and then the grandparents would come and the aunts and uncles and cleaning lady and friends, etc. ... and everyone would come and then we would all get COVID. I remember laughing and saying that I just had a baby and I promised her I had no interest in getting COVID either! I communicated no one was coming to visit us for quite some time. My parents were in Boston, my husband's were in Philadelphia, we had asked our cleaning lady to stop coming, and we were not going to allow any friends or other family to come visit for the foreseeable future. I explained that we would be a little bubble together and fortunately, I convinced her to come.

I left the hospital on day three after just two nights, which is a very quick turnaround for a C-section, but I just wanted to get out of there, and felt that we would be safer at home. My husband came to get us in a taxicab, which was very different from our original plan. My parents were supposed to have come in from Boston, and then my mom would have come to pick us up, having installed the car seat in advance. In contrast to what we had been told about "car seat checks," no one was even looking to see if we had a car seat. We could have walked out of the hospital with the baby and no car seat at all, the hospital was in such a state of disarray. Fortunately, we had purchased the type of car seat that can be used with or without a base, so we were able to secure it in the cab with the seat belt, and we made it safely home.

Almost four years later, our COVID baby is thriving! He is a fun-loving, energetic, intelligent little boy. His first-ever fever was at two and a half years old, probably because we kept him cocooned in our home for so long. He got very used to wearing masks and seeing others in them, to the point that if one of us started to leave the house without one he would remind us that we had forgotten it. But the masks did not slow his language skills down, he is extremely talkative (actually never stops talking) perhaps because we spent so much time at home together reading every single book on our bookshelves. In the fall of 2022, he started school, and I was a bit worried at how he would acclimate given that he had spent so little time in the "outside world," but he has truly flourished, created a huge friend group and community, and we couldn't be prouder.

As a final note, I will say that we welcomed a second son in April 2022. The contrast between the two experiences was night and day. First, Weill Cornell had moved its maternity ward across the street to Alexandra

Cohen, its new space, which is gorgeous, and everyone gets a guaranteed private room. Second, my husband was allowed to stay for the entire time. Third, the nursery was open, and we were encouraged to send our son there so I could rest, and I did get rest! Fourth, the lactation consultants came by nonstop to help, and it made such a difference! I ended up breastfeeding my son for fourteen months and storing up enough milk that he had enough frozen milk for another four months. It was such a pleasure giving birth we were happy to stay there for the full four nights!

The pandemic was a hard time for so many people, some of whom lost lives or loved ones. But the experience of giving birth during the pandemic was a trauma that will stay with me forever. I think that in some ways it will always make me both worry about and appreciate my son in a unique way because of the experience we went through together.

JILL'S STORY

When my husband, Matt, and I decided we were ready to start trying to have a baby, it was a well-thought-out decision. This was going to be our first child and we had a lot of discussions to prepare. We are planners, so we did what we do best, and we made plans. But you know what was not a part of any of those plans? A worldwide pandemic.

Things were already shifting in New York City when I discovered the faint pink line on a stick. New York City, where we lived, and the world were abuzz with panic and uncertainty. Within days of our big news, the city was on lockdown. The school I taught at and my husband's office moved to remote work for the foreseeable future. My always prepared husband suggested we talk to my parents about staying with them in the suburbs for a few weeks, where it felt safer and we'd have some more space. For the record, the "few weeks" became five months. Five months being thirty-five and married and pregnant and sleeping in my childhood bedroom surrounded by my stuffed animals and the Abercrombie shopping bags I'd proudly displayed on my walls as a teenager.

Throughout the entire process, I tried very hard to focus on the positives and maintain a sense of humor about this. At the end of the day, I was grateful to have a healthy pregnancy, and eventually a healthy baby. But being pregnant in a pandemic definitely made you think about things you never thought about before. Like using a portable female urinal funnel to avoid public bathrooms.

Without dwelling too much on the negatives, I think it's important to acknowledge what couples like us lost being first-time parents during this time. We weren't able to share the excitement and celebrate with our friends and family in a normal way. With so many unknowns about how this virus affected pregnant women, we remained incredibly isolated throughout the entire pregnancy. Our friends and family were not with us through this ... they didn't see my body change—as if this entire chunk of time, this major moment in our lives, just didn't exist.

We weren't going into stores, so there was no fun test-driving of strollers while putting our registry together. I did my layette virtually. There were no visitors in the hospital. There was a lot of sadness and anxiety thinking about our parents and siblings not being able to hold their new niece and grandchild. We're both very close to our families, and that is a reality I never could have imagined even considering in a million years.

The hardest part was that my husband could not come to any appointments with me. He heard the baby's heartbeat for the first time on the phone, sitting in our parked car outside of my ob-gyn's office. I'd FaceTime him during the Q and A portion of my exams, but he never actually met any of the doctors at the practice and didn't before the day our daughter was delivered. Thankfully, he was at least with me for that. I know other women who gave birth in the spring of 2020 where this was not the case.

I'd FaceTime him so he could see the blurry screen during my sonograms. But so much of his participation in this process was remotely from the car. This was particularly hard when we hit bumps in the road in the pregnancy, like when I had spotting at eleven weeks and had to make an emergency appointment to make sure we hadn't lost the baby or when my fluid levels dropped in my last weeks, moving up my C-section before its scheduled date. I completely understand why it was the case, and I am grateful that my doctors were taking every precaution to keep mamas-to-be and their developing babies safe. But there's really no way around it—it was really hard for us both.

All of this, coupled with the state of the world and our country often left me feeling like, "What are we bringing a child into?!" But there were positives of being pregnant in a pandemic too. Pregnancy equals feeling tired all the time, especially at the beginning, so it was pretty amazing to be at home and be able to easily rest when necessary. I had more time with my husband than I ever would have if we had not been in this situation. It was pretty special to have so much time just the two of us, before we became a unit of three. It also forced a pivot to a virtual model in my business that ultimately changed my life for the better and likely wouldn't have happened otherwise.

Obviously, I knew that becoming a parent was a huge responsibility that would involve making a lot of decisions and choices. But having to make these calls and ask ourselves, "Is this safe for my child?" before doing every single thing ... establishing our "rules" but not wanting to dictate what others are comfortable with, trying to navigate and make decisions in the name of her safety in a situation that is constantly evolving. It was so hard and so draining. What risks were worth taking? Which were not? The stakes felt so high. Because they were so high.

There were so many milestones in my daughter's first year that we couldn't share with many people we love in person. So many friends and family members that didn't meet her until much later than I'd ever thought would be the case. So many things I'd imagined doing with her in her first year that we didn't do.

I know so many of us experienced that in our own ways, being pregnant and then parenting in a pandemic, making our own tough calls. Because of my work in the parenting space, I was able to connect with other pregnant women and then, eventually, other new parents virtually. Hearing their stories and sharing our feelings and unique struggles and experiences brought a lot of comfort. And despite the challenges, it felt easier when you realized you weren't alone.

CONCLUSION

The women whose experiences filled these pages shared their inspiring stories of pregnancy and childbirth during the early days of the COVID-19 pandemic in a way that shows true vulnerability and strength. It is my hope that their stories and fortitude will serve as a bright light for other women who go through a dark time in pregnancy/birth—whether it be a pandemic or other crisis.

Feeling supported can encourage strength. When going through something difficult, feeling that you are not alone and that someone else has been through something similar can help inspire courage and strength. Who couldn't use more courage and strength during difficult times?

Feeling heard can facilitate healing. After experiencing a traumatic event like a global pandemic, recognizing what was abnormal, hard, and difficult, along with anything positive and sharing it can help in processing the experience. This can potentially reduce the lingering effects of trauma.

I hope this book has provided a platform for women to be supported, to feel heard, and to heal. **Strength is in community**.

ACKNOWLEDGMENTS

When I sat down to write this there was not a second of hesitation before knowing who I needed to extend gratitude toward first. Thank you to the most incredible human being I know, my child. You make every single day better by being in the world. Being pregnant during the pandemic gave me the idea for this book—a collection of stories to inspire strength in women who will go through a similar experience in the future, and to allow women who have gone through this unique experience the opportunity to share and be heard. Without you, my baby, there is a good chance this book would never have been written.

I am immensely grateful to the women who formed the community on which this book stands. I have so much gratitude for the women who shared their important personal stories to build this beautiful collection. Your vulnerability and strength make up the fibers of this book.

I am also so thankful to the women who spread the word about my submission requests for this book, which helped to build a great foundation for this project. Jessica Hill, founder of the Parenthood Collective, and Ashley Comegys, founder of Raised to Empower. You both "got" this project from the start and seem to truly understand the meaning of strength in community. A thank-you is much deserved to the Breastfeeding Center for Greater Washington and the Brookside Mothers' Association for sharing my request for submissions with your community too. Jill Lerman, who fosters a sense of community and support among mothers every day as a play consultant with her company Jillybeans NYC, thank you for sharing your story and graciously sharing my request with your community.

I want to express gratitude to those along the way who offered words of encouragement when I would first tell them about the project. The first reactions to an idea have an impact. Shirley Bergin, thank you for leading by example when it comes to the importance of real dialogue about pregnancy and childbirth and for your support. Emma Moylan, thank you for your eagle eye.

I must express my gratitude to you, the reader. Reading these stories allows the women who went through these experiences to be heard. It also increases the likelihood that these stories will serve as a source of strength and encouragement to women in the future. Please share the book and the message it embodies.

Last, to come full circle, thank you to Anita Sampson (age one hundred in 2020) whose words gave me a boost of strength during the pandemic. Sharing your own mother's (and your) pandemic story provided needed hope for an eventual return to normalcy during the early days of the pandemic—at a time in which life felt so surreal to myself and many others.

APPENDIX

Stay-at-Home Orders Issued in All or Parts of the State (USA)
*no stay-at-home order statewide or in parts of the state
**partial

Alabama April 4, 2020

Alaska March 28, 2020

Arizona March 31, 2020

Arkansas *

California March 19, 2020

Colorado March 26, 2020

Connecticut March 23, 2020

Delaware March 24, 2020

District of Columbia April 1, 2020

Florida April 3, 2020

Georgia April 3, 2020

Hawaii March 25, 2020

Idaho March 25, 2020

Illinois March 21, 2020

Indiana March 24, 2020

Iowa *

Kansas March 30, 2020

Kentucky March 26, 2020

Louisiana March 23, 2020

Maine April 2, 2020

Maryland March 30, 2020

Massachusetts March 24, 2020

Michigan March 24, 2020

Minnesota March 27, 2020

Mississippi April 3, 2020

Missouri April 6, 2020

Montana March 28, 2020

Nebraska *

Nevada April 1, 2020

New Hampshire March 27, 2020

New Jersey March 24, 2020

New Mexico Mach 24, 2020

New York March 22, 2020

North Carolina March 30, 2020

North Dakota *

Ohio March 23, 2020

Oklahoma ** *Partial* March 28, 2020, Oklahoma City and Tulsa

Oregon March 23, 2020

Pennsylvania April 1, 2020

Rhode Island March 28, 2020

South Carolina April 6, 2020

South Dakota *

Tennessee March 31, 2020

Texas April 2, 2020

Utah ** *Partial* March 27, 2020, Summit County March 30, 2020, Salt Lake County/Wasatch County April 1, 2020, Davis County

Vermont March 25, 2020

Virginia March 30, 2020

Washington March 23, 2020

West Virginia March 24, 2020

Wisconsin March 25, 2020

Wyoming ** *Partial* March 28, 2020, Jackson

NOTES

[i] Ozbay, Fatih, et al. "Social Support and Resilience to Stress: From Neurobiology to Clinical Practice." *Psychiatry (Edgmont (Pa.: Township))*, vol. 4, no. 5, 1 May 2007, pp. 35–40, https://pubmed.ncbi.nlm.nih.gov/20806028/.

[ii] Schnall, Simone, et al. "Social Support and the Perception of Geographical Slant." *Journal of Experimental Social Psychology*, vol. 44, no. 5, 2008, pp. 1246–1255., https://doi.org/10.1016/j.jesp.2008.04.011.

[iii] Born in Quarantine. (2020, May 10). Facebook. *Television.*

[iv] Marani, Marco, et al. "Intensity and Frequency of Extreme Novel Epidemics." *Proceedings of the National Academy of Sciences*, vol. 118, no. 35, 31 Aug. 2021, www.pnas.org/content/118/35/e2105482118, 10.1073/pnas.2105482118.

[v] Alison Hermann, M. D. (2021, February 1). *Meeting maternal mental health needs during the COVID-19 pandemic.* JAMA Psychiatry. https://jamanetwork.com/journals/jamapsychiatry/fullarticle/2768028#yvp200030r1

[vi] Sarah Meaney, et al. "The impact of COVID-19 on pregnant womens' experiences and perceptions of antenatal maternity care, social support, and stress-reduction strategies." *Women and Birth*, vol. 35, no. 3, 2022, pp. 307–316, https://www.sciencedirect.com/science/article/pii/S1871519221000792

[vii] Boserup, B., McKenney, M., & Elkbuli, A. (2020, December). *Alarming trends in US domestic violence during the COVID-19 pandemic.* The American journal of emergency medicine. https://www.ncbi.nlm.nih.gov/pmc/articles/PMC7195322/

[viii] King, L. S., Feddoes, D. E., Kirshenbaum, J. S., Humphreys, K. L., & Gotlib, I. H. (2021, March 30). *Pregnancy during the pandemic: The impact of covid-19-related stress on risk for prenatal depression.* Psychological medicine. https://www.ncbi.nlm.nih.gov/pmc/articles/PMC8047399/

[ix] Kotlar, B., Gerson, E., Petrillo, S., Langer, A., & Tiemeier, H. (2021, January 18). *The impact of the COVID-19 pandemic on maternal and Perinatal Health: A scoping review – reproductive health.* BioMed Central. https://reproductive-health-journal.biomedcentral.com/articles/10.1186/s12978-021-01070-6

[x] Karageorge, E. X. (2020, September). *Covid-19 recession is tougher on women: Monthly labor review.* U.S. Bureau of Labor Statistics. https://www.bls.gov/opub/mlr/2020/beyond-bls/covid-19-recession-is-tougher-on-women.htm

[xi] Chivers, B. R., Garad, R. M., Boyle, J. A., Skouteris, H., Teede, H. J., & Harrison, C. L. (2020, September 7). *Perinatal distress during COVID-19: Thematic analysis of an online Parenting Forum.* Journal of medical Internet research. https://www.ncbi.nlm.nih.gov/pmc/articles/PMC7481017/

[xii] Mervosh, S., Lu, D., & Swales, V. (2020, March 24). *See which states and cities have told residents to stay at home.* The New York Times. https://www.nytimes.com/interactive/2020/us/coronavirus-stay-at-home-order.html

[xiii] Bringé, A. (2022, November 9). *Council post: The rise of athleisure in the fashion industry and what it means for brands.* Forbes. https://www.forbes.com/sites/forbescommunicationscouncil/2021/05/03/the-rise-of-athleisure-in-the-fashion-industry-and-what-it-means-for-brands/?sh=2ebc20813ae0

[xiv] Prideaux, E. (2021, February 3). *How to heal the 'mass trauma' of covid-19.* BBC Future. https://www.bbc.com/future/article/20210203-after-the-covid-19-pandemic-how-will-we-heal

[xv] "Stress in America 2023: A Nation Recovering from Collective Trauma." *American Psychological Association*, American Psychological Association, www.apa.org/news/press/releases/stress/2023/collective-trauma-recovery.

www.ingramcontent.com/pod-product-compliance
Lightning Source LLC
Chambersburg PA
CBHW032102040426
42449CB00007B/1152